Dear Me...
Al...

D1553549

Thank You for

AROMATHERAPY
recipes for beauty, health,
and well-being

Victoria H. Edwards

a WONDER FILLED
stay - as usual ☺
Hope this book
brings you Happiness.
I Love You,
Shakti

The mission of Storey Publishing is to serve our customers by publishing practical information that encourages personal independence in harmony with the environment.

Edited by Deborah Balmuth and Karen Levy
Cover design by Wendy Palitz
Anatomical illustrations by Alison Kolesar
Text design and production by Susan Bernier

Printed in the United States by Lake Book
10 9 8 7 6 5 4 3 2 1

ISBN 1-58017-891-X

In very simple terms, aromatherapy is the therapeutic use of pure essential oils to improve the health and balance of the skin, the body, the mind, and the soul.

Squeeze a lavender head or a sage leaf and smell your fingers. That aroma is the result of volatile oils, released by the bursting of tiny glands in the plant material. These volatile oils represent the radiant energy of the sun, translated by the plant into a chemical form. If you look at the same plant through a microscope, you will see the little pouches where these chemicals, the volatile oils, are stored. Although we

Information and Cautions

Most of the ingredients mentioned in this book can be found in natural-food or health-food stores. Natural product and herbal mail-order suppliers may also have them.

Use caution in handling pure essential oils. Because they are highly concentrated, they can burn or cause adverse skin reactions. Most essential oils should be diluted in a base oil before application to the skin. Always use a dropper when measuring essential oils, and do not use more than recommended; more can be dangerous, not better. Never use essential oils near the eyes. Consult your doctor before using essential oils if you are pregnant. Do not ingest essential oils, and avoid sun exposure while using them. Keep all ingredients out of the reach of children and pets.

When using any ingredient for the first time, do a patch test. Apply a bit of the ingredient to the inside of your arm and allow it to remain for 24 hours. If you see any signs of allergic response — redness, itching, or other skin irritation — discontinue use immediately.

don't yet fully understand the role these essential oils play in the drama of plants' life cycles, they have played a role throughout the development of human culture.

The quantity and quality of the essential oils that a plant produces depend on many things. Just as soil, elevation, and weather conditions; genus and species; horticulture; processing; and handling all influence the ultimate quality of a fine wine, so essential oils for therapeutic use vary according to the plants' conditions of growth.

What Are Essential Oils?

Essential oils are a cocktail of molecules with names like esters, terpenes, alcohols, phenols, aldehydes, ketones, ethers, and sesquiterpenes, along with a myriad of other chemicals. These constituent parts have various properties. Some are anti-inflammatory, some antifungal, some antiviral, mucolytic, or bactericidal. All are antiseptic in varying degrees, and all are volatile. Essential oils naturally fall into three groups. The most volatile essential oils, known as *top notes* in the perfume industry, are those that evaporate most quickly. These oils tend to have an uplifting and invigorating action. Essential oils that have a lower volatility, and thus evaporate slowly, are known to perfumers as *bass notes*. These oils are most often used therapeutically for their calming and sedating action. And essential oils with a medium range of volatility, known as *middle notes* in perfumery, act to stimulate and regulate the main body systems.

Natural oils do not cause side effects when used properly. Essential oils have the power to relax the nervous system, stimulate the circulation, lift depression, reduce inflammation, and ease aches and pains. They can balance emotions by establishing harmony between the mind and body and lifting the conscious mind to the higher self. The aroma of an essential oil is sensed by the olfactory nerve located in the back of the nose and is carried to the brain, where it has its effect — perhaps stimulating or calming, perhaps imparting feelings of well-being and harmony to the whole self.

Oils can also penetrate the skin's surface, and their benefits for the skin are profound. Essential oils can revitalize and rejuvenate skin of all ages and are especially helpful for problems such as acne, eczema, psoriasis, burns, scars, and even some skin cancers.

A professional aromatherapy treatment is usually combined with massage. Therapeutic and healing in itself, massage has magnified effects when combined with aromatherapy. Massage can make us feel comforted and secure, because touch is an extension of our earliest memories; when combined with the appropriate essential oils, the benefits for mind and body are considerable.

Although many of the effects of essential oils have been proven through scientific research, their most profound healing qualities can only be observed. The effects of aromas on the psyche, along with their subtler contribution to prevention of illness, are difficult to measure. But aromatherapy is one of the oldest healing arts known to humankind.

The Origins of Aromatherapy

The origins of aromatherapy lie hidden in the folds of time. Humankind's earliest written documents record the use of plant oils for their healing and aesthetic properties. Ointments, oils, infusions, poultices, and incenses were all made from plants, and they were the only medicines known until the late 19th century.

Ancient healers were holistic. They regarded healing as a transcendent art. From the same plants they used to heal the body, they derived perfumes to uplift the spirit, and they recognized these two actions as different aspects of the same unifying plant energy. In contrast, modern science seeks to compartmentalize, and it works to identify and separate plants' active constituents.

How Essential Oils Are Made

Although the term *essential oil* is commonly used to refer to any oil that has been extracted from a plant, a "true" essential oil is one that has been collected through steam distillation. The French consider steam-distilled oils to be the only true essential oils and the only ones worthy of use in aromatherapy.

Using Aromatherapy

There are countless ways to use aromatherapy in your own life. Essential oils can be applied directly to the skin as part of massage, reflexology, or meridian treatment. They can be dispersed in bath water, inhaled, or diffused into the atmosphere of a room. Specific oils affect specific systems throughout the body. You can target these various systems if you know how to select an essential oil for its particular properties and how to select an effective and efficient means of delivery in each case.

Aromatherapy Through the Day

By incorporating aromatherapy into your daily routine, you can enjoy the natural health benefits of essential oils and enhance previously humdrum activities and routines.

Imagine waking to the invigorating scent of rosemary and basil drifting gently past your nose. It's not hard to achieve: Load a diffuser with a wake-up blend and use an automatic timer. In your morning shower, give your body an energizing loofah scrub with a solution of thyme, savory, and tea tree oil. Follow your shower with a quick toweling, and then lock the residual moisture into your skin with a custom-designed body oil blend. You might add a few drops of tea tree oil to the toothpaste on your toothbrush to help prevent gum disease and tooth decay.

On your way to work, place a tissue moistened with a drop of lavender essential oil on the dashboard of your car to smooth out the drive. Along with your lipstick, carry a vial of peppermint oil: A drop on your tongue throughout the day will keep your breath fresh and help you stay alert. Before an important meeting, you might place a drop of rose oil on your tongue. It will give you confidence and create a loving atmosphere as the scent of rose is broadcast with your presentation. On your drive home, a little clary sage on a tissue placed on your dashboard will help you unwind and cope with rush-hour traffic.

Later, an evening bath with chamomile, neroli, and marjoram will ensure a restful sleep. Or if you are cold, you might prefer a warming bath with black pepper, myrrh, sandalwood, Peru balsam, and ginger — ahhh, another aromatic day!

What if you wake up feeling miserable? When everything hurts, or when you've got the blues, cramps, or a headache, cancel your plans and take a hot steaming bath with eucalyptus, geranium, clary sage, and juniper. Make yourself a pot of herbal tea and snuggle up in a warm bathrobe. You're sure to feel better soon.

Effective Application Techniques
for Particular Body Systems

Essential Oil Application	Internal Organs and Systems Affected
Bath or spa therapy; massage and frictions; "aroma glows"	Works energetically on organ meridians
Algae, seaweed, and thalassotherapy; herbal aromatic body wraps; poultices	Endocrine system
Inhalation with diffusers	Respiratory, pulmonary systems; neurochemical responses
Internal uses; douches and boluses; suppositories	Digestive, eliminative, and oral systems
Subtle work; essences, crystals, color lights; homeopathy	Emotional responses

Airborne Scent

One of the miracles of aromatherapy is its absolute simplicity. Just a whiff of the right oil can adjust your attitude, clarify your thinking, steady your resolve, even ease your pain. Lavender is often in my pocket for brief inhalations whenever stress is beating me down. A whiff of lemon invariably clears my head and refreshes my thought processes. Inhalations are a practical way to incorporate aromatherapy into your day.

Jet Lag Inhalation

  5 drops bay laurel essential oil
  5 drops geranium essential oil
  5 drops lavender essential oil

Combine the oils in a small glass vial with a tight stopper.
To use: Carry a vial in your pocket or purse while traveling. Sniff periodically throughout the day to forestall the exhaustion and brain fog of jet lag.

Stress-Buster #1

Stress wreaks havoc on the immune system. This blend will help give the system a healthy boost.

- 5 drops niaouli essential oil
- 5 drops ravensara essential oil

Combine the oils in a small glass vial with a tight stopper.
To use: Carry a vial in your pocket or purse and sniff periodically throughout the day.

Stress-Buster #2

This is a very calming blend.

- 2 drops Roman chamomile essential oil
- 5 drops lavender essential oil
- 34 drops ylang-ylang essential oil

Combine the oils in a small glass vial with a tight stopper.
To use: Carry a vial in your pocket or purse and sniff periodically throughout the day.

Media Overload

  3 drops nutmeg essential oil
  5 drops clove essential oil
 10 drops sandalwood essential oil

Combine the oils in a small glass vial with a tight stopper.
To use: Carry a vial in your pocket or purse or keep it at
your desk. If you're working at a computer terminal for
extended periods, sniff periodically throughout the day.

The Aromatic Diffuser

There are many ways of scenting an environment. Incense
has been used to deliver scent for thousands of years. More
recently candle burners, simmering potpourri pots, and
lightbulb rings have all become popular methods of dispersing scent. These methods are aesthetically pleasing but
are not the best choices for aromatherapy. Commercial
incense and potpourris are often rounded out with synthetic scents; their purity is unreliable. Additionally, incense

smoke may transmit harsh, and even carcinogenic, chemicals along with its pleasing aroma. Candle burners and lightbulb rings can overheat delicate essential oils, changing their chemical makeup.

Diffusers act quite differently. Without altering or heating oils, they disperse them into the environment via an air-jet pump connected to a glass bell. A nebulizer within the glass bell diffuses a fine mist of negatively charged, scented ions into the atmosphere, much the same way that nature spreads fragrance.

The aromatic diffuser first appeared in Paris in 1960, when Dr. Bidault demonstrated the germicidal action of aromatic essences on tuberculosis, whooping cough, and influenza. His clinical observations indicated that disinfection of the air surrounding a patient had a therapeutic preventive effect. At the University of Paris School of Pharmacy, students tested his theories by collecting samples of air from an urban factory, the forest of Fontainebleau on the out-

Diffuser Blends for De-Stressing

- **To ease colds and flu:** Oregano, lavender, eucalyptus, thyme, clove, cinnamon, peppermint
- **To calm:** Lavender, marjoram, geranium, chamomile
- **To dispel nervous tension:** Lemon, orange, neroli
- **To promote meditation:** Clary sage, fir, cedar
- **To counter depression:** Bergamot, geranium, clary sage

skirts of the city, and a Parisian apartment. By diffusing various essential oils into sealed chambers containing the air samples, they were able to validate the effectiveness of the essential oils against airborne bacteria and molds.

The modern aromatic diffuser is a natural alternative to aerosol deodorizers and chemical air fresheners. A diffuser is a safe and convenient method of dispersing essential oils throughout a home, school, or workplace.

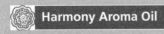

Harmony Aroma Oil

This formula can be adjusted to suit your particular emotional and physical needs. You may want to create all three of the versions listed below so you'll have the appropriate one on hand when needed. *Caution:* These formulas are for inhalation only. Do not apply directly to the skin; they may cause irritation.

    1 tablespoon pure, unrefined almond, jojoba,
      or hazelnut oil
    1 of the following blends

Calming Blend: For excess stress, restlessness, or trouble sleeping, or if the weather outside is cold and dry, add ½ teaspoon lavender, ½ teaspoon neroli, ½ teaspoon clary sage, and ½ teaspoon bergamot essential oils.

Cooling Blend: For irritability, impatience, fiery disposition, or chaos, or if the weather is hot and sticky and your skin is sensitive and itchy, add ½ teaspoon lavender, ½ teaspoon jasmine, ½ teaspoon Roman chamomile, and ½ teaspoon spearmint essential oils.

Stimulating Blend: If you're feeling slow and lethargic, in need of an energetic lift, and maybe a bit congested, or if the weather is dreary, cool, and damp, add ½ teaspoon cinnamon, ½ teaspoon orange, ½ teaspoon ginger, and ½ teaspoon cypress essential oils.

Combine the almond, jojoba, or hazelnut oil with the blend of your choice in a 2-ounce, dark-colored glass bottle and cap tightly. The blend needs one week to synergize and develop, so shake your formula vigorously twice daily for seven days. After one week, place a few drops on a soft handkerchief or tissue and inhale the comforting herbal aroma as needed. The aroma can also be inhaled directly from the bottle.

By using a diffuser, it is possible to dispense a therapeutic aromatherapy treatment to a number of people simultaneously. It is an excellent way of purifying the environment as well as administering the uplifting, rejuvenating, or relaxing effects of selected oils or blends to a group.

In the home environment, the therapeutic effects of diffused oils on the respiratory system are especially helpful during the cold and flu season, because the diffuser destroys airborne bacteria. When outside air is polluted, a diffuser can help create a safe, peaceful, and uplifting atmosphere indoors.

Relaxation Blend

  5 drops petitgrain essential oil
10 drops mandarin essential oil
20 drops lavender *(Lavandula angustifolia)* essential oil

Combine the oils in a dark glass vial and shake to mix.
To use: Use in a diffuser to encourage relaxation.

Asthma with Nervousness and Allergies Blend

1 teaspoon mandarin essential oil
1 teaspoon tarragon essential oil
1 teaspoon rosemary 'verbenon' essential oil

Combine the oils in a dark glass vial with a tight stopper and shake to mix. **To use:** Use in a diffuser during asthma flare-ups. Or carry in a small glass vial to be sniffed frequently throughout the day.

Detoxification Blend

1 teaspoon everlasting essential oil
1 teaspoon rose geranium essential oil
2 teaspoons lemon essential oil

Combine the oils in a dark glass vial and shake to mix.
To use: Use this blend in a diffuser when detoxifying the body or working to break a smoking, alcohol, or other drug habit. This blend can also be carried with you, or kept in your desk, to be sniffed directly from the glass vial throughout the day.

Meditation Blend #1

2 drops cistus essential oil
2 drops clove essential oil
2 drops rose essential oil
4 drops myrrh essential oil
5 drops sandalwood essential oil
10 drops frankincense essential oil

Combine the oils in a dark glass vial and shake well.
To use: Add to a diffuser and use to support and enhance meditation.

Meditation Blend #2

2 drops cistus essential oil
4 drops vetiver essential oil
5 drops fir essential oil
10 drops clary sage essential oil
20 drops cedarwood essential oil

Combine the oils in a dark glass vial and shake well.
To use: Diffuse to support and enhance meditation.

Topical Applications

Most of us see the skin as a natural barrier. We imagine that our skin not only holds us in, but also keeps everything else out. We imagine that if our skin is unbroken, we present an impermeable surface to the world and are immune to the chemical stew of our environment. But the skin, the body's largest organ, is not at all impermeable. Acting more like a very fine sieve, our skin "breathes." As it inhales, it absorbs fine traces of whatever is on its surface; as it exhales, it excretes chemicals as fine components of sweat and sloughed-off skin cells.

The outer skin, made up of about 30 layers of cells, is called the epidermis. We shed dead skin cells every day. As the top layer of the skin dies off, a new layer is generated at the base. But as the skin ages, this process of cellular reproduction slows down. If the top layers are not sloughed off, the formation of new skin cells is slowed even further, and the complexion becomes tired and muddy-looking.

In 1968, researchers demonstrated the permeability of the human skin by attaching radioactive "tags" to chemicals incorporated into cosmetic preparations. The preparations were applied to the skin of human volunteers, and the tagged chemicals were later identified in the volunteers' waste products. When I read about this study it dramatically changed my attitude about the ingredients I was putting on my skin.

I learned that when essential oils are placed on the skin they are absorbed rapidly. In as little as 5 to 20 minutes an essential oil, when applied topically, makes its way into the bloodstream, is carried through to the lungs, and is exhaled with every breath. Essential oils are also eliminated through the skin, released in sweat through the pores, and released in urine through the bladder. As the essential oil makes its journey through the various body systems, the body's many tissues and organs obtain benefit from its healing action.

Sleepytime Balm

So simple to make, yet so effective. This balm is gentle enough to safely pacify even the most irritable, restless infant.

- ¼ cup all-vegetable shortening (room temperature)
- 2 drops essential oil of ylang-ylang
- 10 drops essential oil of orange
- 1 drop essential oil of vanilla (optional)

Combine all ingredients in a small bowl and whip together using a small spatula or whisk. Store in a 2-ounce plastic or glass jar in a dry, cool place for up to four months. **To use:** Apply a dab to your temples after cleansing your face and just prior to bedtime. Use daily, if desired.

The Seven-Step Facial

Practiced weekly, this facial-care program will cleanse and revitalize a dull complexion, relax the mind, and nourish the soul. If you open yourself to the present moment and the aromatic, soothing touch that these gifts from nature — herbs, flowers, essential oils, and other ingredients — can offer, you can truly luxuriate in this spa experience.

1. Cleanse. Use the mild soap or cleanser of your choice.

2. Exfoliate. Keep a jar of homemade cleansing grains on hand — equal parts oatmeal, cornmeal, and ground almonds. Take about 1 tablespoon of the grains in the palm of your hand, add a little warm water to form a paste, and gently scrub your face and neck. Allow the grains to set on your face for a few minutes, then rinse with warm water or rub off gently with your fingertips.

3. Steam. Heat 2 quarts of water to a simmer and pour into a large basin or bowl. Add 2 to 4 drops of an essential oil of your choice (see chart at right). Lean your face over the steaming water and drape a bath towel over the back of your head, forming a tent to capture the steam. Be careful not to burn yourself. Relax and let the fragrant steam engulf your head for 5 to 10 minutes.

Choosing Essential Oils for Your Skin Type

Skin Type	Recommended Essential Oils
Acned or congested	Thyme (sweet), neroli, bergamot, tea tree, spike lavender, sandalwood
Normal	Lemon, jasmine, rose, lavender, chamomile
Dehydrated	Carrot, rosemary 'verbenon', neroli, sandalwood, inula, everlasting
Oily	Melissa, lemon, lemongrass, basil, eucalyptus (E. radiata), camphor
Mature or wrinkled	Myrrh, frankincense, angelica, cistus, spikenard, violet, galbanum
Fragile, sensitive, or allergic	Bulgarian rose, blue artemis, blue chamomile, lavender

4. **Massage.** Gently pat your face dry — don't rub it. Choose a facial oil blend from the recipes listed on the following pages and sprinkle a few drops into your palms. Rub

your palms together and massage lightly over your face. Starting at the base of your neck, massage up the throat in a sweeping motion to your chin. From the corners of your nose, sweep under the cheekbones and up to your temples. Smoothing across your forehead, continue around your ears to the back of the neck, then down over your neck, shoulders, and chest.

5. Mask. Choose one of the healing clay masks on pages 29–31. Apply to your entire face and neck, avoiding your lips and the area around the eyes. Apply thickly to any areas congested with pimples or blackheads. Leave on for 20 minutes and then remove with a moistened washcloth.

6. Tone. Apply the toner of your choice (see pages 33–35) to clarify your complexion, close your pores, and remove any residual clay.

7. Moisturize. Top off your facial with a light application of a moisturizer or facial oil blend. In a few hours, your face will be glowing with health and vitality.

Facial Oils

Facial oils soothe and nourish the delicate skin of the face. They seal the skin, helping it retain precious moisture and providing protection from surface contaminants. They are also an important component of facial massage — by reducing friction, they prevent stretching and wrinkling of the skin. The delicate scent of the essential oils can be quite relaxing and will linger with you through the day.

Sensitive or Inflamed Skin Lotion

2 drops chamomile essential oil
2 drops neroli essential oil
5 drops bois de rose essential oil
7 drops sandalwood essential oil
1 ounce hazelnut oil

Combine all ingredients in a small, dark glass bottle; shake to mix.

To use: After cleansing and toning, place a few drops in the palms of your hands and massage lightly over your face.

Oily-Skin Lotion

  5 drops cypress essential oil
10 drops niaouli essential oil
  1 ounce hazelnut oil

Combine all ingredients in a small, dark glass bottle; shake to mix. **To use:** After cleansing and toning, place a few drops in the palms of your hands and massage lightly over your face.

Aging-Skin Lotion

This wonderful formula supports cellular regeneration.

1 teaspoon lavender essential oil
1 teaspoon rose geranium essential oil
1 teaspoon rosemary 'borneol' essential oil
1 teaspoon sage essential oil

Combine all ingredients in a small, dark glass bottle; shake to mix. **To use:** After cleansing and toning, place a few drops in the palms of your hands and massage lightly over your face and neck.

Moisturizing Lotion

 3 drops vetiver essential oil
 5 drops orange essential oil
10 drops lavender essential oil
 1 ounce almond oil

Combine all ingredients in a small, dark glass bottle; shake to mix. **To use:** After cleansing and toning, place a few drops in the palms of your hands and massage lightly over your face and neck.

Clay Masks

Clay is one of the oldest of all skin treatments. It was even used by the women of ancient Egypt as they bathed along the banks of the Nile. It contains an abundance of silica and other mineral salts. Silica is a natural mineral that can take many forms and acts as a carrier of catalysts in chemical reactions. It is present in sand and glass and is found in the human body wherever hard edges appear, such as the skin, nails, and hair.

Clay is a balancer and revitalizer. When applied to the skin as a mask, oxidation and circulation are accelerated, defensive functions are stimulated, and body temperature is raised.

Clay has certain little quirks that are important to know about. Dry clay powder can be stored easily. It is often sold in paper packaging, and no harm will come if dry clay is stored in plastic. However, as soon as water is introduced, the clay is activated; from this point it should come into contact only with organic materials. This means mixing and storing in glass or ceramic vessels. Wet clay doesn't agree with plastic, and combining clays with metals can set off unpredictable and undesirable chemical changes.

Use wooden spoons or chopsticks for mixing and stirring, and make sure the water you are using is pure. You don't want to apply a clay mask with bacteria growing in it! Distilled water is your best assurance of purity, but a reliable hydrosol (see pages 36–41) or spring water can enhance the action of a clay mask. Measure your dry clay into a ceramic bowl and stir in enough water or hydrosol to form a soft paste. Add a few drops of an essential oil of your choice (use 3 to 5 drops per ounce of wet clay) and mix thoroughly. Apply to your entire face and neck, avoiding your lips and the area around the eyes. Leave the mask on until it is dry, and then wash off with warm water or scrub off for an exfoliation treatment.

Use only healing clays found in health-food stores. The type of clay used for ceramics is not recommended.

• **Green clay** is an excellent all-purpose clay for healing and cleansing.

• **Rose clay** is highly absorbent and thus more drying. It makes a wonderful cleansing mask.

• **White clay** is very light and pure; used in its dry form, it is an excellent base for body powders.

• **Yellow clay** contains sulfur compounds. It's used to make clay packs to promote the healing of broken bones as well as to treat bone pain, sprains, and muscle aches and strains.

Astringents and Toners

Astringents and toners are essential to any facial cleansing routine. They invigorate the complexion, remove traces of soap, close the pores, and quickly restore the skin's protective acid mantle (pH level).

Aroma Friction

Using this blend with loofah scrubs is energizing and toning.

    3 drops savory essential oil
    5 drops thyme essential oil
   12 drops MQV essential oil
    3 ounces distilled/spring water

Combine all ingredients in a spray bottle; shake to mix.
To use: To stimulate circulation, spray onto a loofah and scrub briskly over your body before or after a shower. Stimulate your meridians by working from foot to groin, from fingertips to chest, and up the backs of your legs.

Cucumber Toner

This is a wonderful formula for clarifying the complexion. Use it to feel crisp and clean during hot and muggy weather.

½ cucumber, diced
2 drops rosemary essential oil
15 tablespoons lavender hydrosol
1 ounce witch hazel

1. Combine all ingredients in a blender and blend until the cucumber is liquified.
2. Strain through a coffee filter or cheesecloth. Put in a dark glass bottle with a lid and store in the refrigerator. **To use:** Apply to the face and neck after cleansing.

 Keep It Fresh

Any recipe that calls for fresh fruit or vegetable products will keep for only 2 or 3 days, even when refrigerated. Adding lemon juice or a few drops of rosemary essential oil will help preserve it. Make only in a quantity that you will use quickly.

Herbal Toner

- 1 cup distilled or spring water
- 1 ounce witch hazel
- 2 tablespoons *each* of the following herbs (dried): nettles, fennel, coltsfoot, marsh mallow, benzoin gum, comfrey, calendula, peppermint, orange blossoms, eucalyptus, chamomile, lavender, elderberries, lemon peel
- 12 drops lavender essential oil
- 12 drops lemon essential oil
- 1 ounce aloe vera gel
- 1 ounce glycerin

1. Combine the water and witch hazel in a small saucepan and heat to a simmer. Remove from the heat.

2. Add the dried herbs and allow to steep for 10 minutes.

3. Add the lavender and lemon essential oils to the herbal mixture and stir.

4. Strain the liquid through a cheesecloth to remove herbs. Add the aloe vera and glycerin.

5. Use a small funnel to pour the liquid into a dark glass bottle. Seal with a lid.

To use: Apply to the face with a cotton ball or pad to refresh the complexion and remove any residual soap or cleanser.

Body Tonic

This is a wonderful tonic for skin that needs firming.

    2 drops sage essential oil
   10 drops rosemary essential oil
   12 drops lavender essential oil
    1 teaspoon glycerin or solubol
    4 ounces rose water

1. Dissolve the essential oils in the glycerin or solubol.
2. Add to the rose water in a spray bottle; shake to mix.
To use: Use as a body spray, after bathing, or as an invigorating pick-me-up.

Brisk Toner

   10 drops lemon essential oil
   1½ teaspoons apple cider vinegar
    4 ounces distilled water

Combine all ingredients in a dark glass bottle. Shake well.
To use: Apply to the face and neck after cleansing.

Hydrosols

Hydrosols (also called flower waters and hydrolats) are by-products of essential oil production, created during distillation. The waters used in the distillation process become naturally scented and impregnated with the plants' subtle water-soluble properties. Flower waters have been produced and used in cooking and cosmetics since ancient times in

 Types of Hydrosols

Herbal hydrosols make excellent toners and skin refreshers. Those currently produced and commonly available include:

Bulgarian rose	Lemon verbena	Peppermint
Eucalyptus	Linden	Rose geranium
Everlasting	Melissa	Rosemary
Hyssop	Moroc rose	Rosemary 'verbenon'
Inula	Myrtle	Thyme
Lavandin	Neroli	Turkish rose
Lavender	Orange blossom	

the Middle East, Tunisia, Egypt, and India. Jeanne Rose, executive director of the Aromatic Plant Project, has popularized herbal hydrosols in North America. She notes that *herbal hydrosols* is a more accurate term than *flower waters*, as many of the waters are made from leaves, bark, or other parts of plants.

The process of performing steam distillation using aromatic plants creates two distinct but complementary products: the essential oil and the hydrosol. Following the cooling of the aromatic gas, the oil-soluble components separate from the water. As they separate, they pass on part of their qualities and a small percentage of themselves: Approximately 2 to 10 percent of the essential oil ends up in the hydrosol.

Hydrosols present themselves as perfect companions to alternative health therapies such as phytotherapy and homeopathy, and they are excellent for people who are too sensitive to use essential oils.

Choosing the Right Hydrosol

Skin Type/Use	Recommended Hydrosols
Normal skin	Neroli, rose, lavender, rosemary
Dry skin	Rosemary, orange blossom, rose
Oily skin	Melissa, lemon verbena, inula
Mature skin	Rose geranium, everlasting, rose
Eye compress	Myrtle, elder flower, chamomile

Applying Hydrosols

All hydrosols can be applied directly to the skin with a cotton ball or pad, or by misting 10 to 12 inches from the face with an atomizer that has a fine mist.

Hydrosols are perfect during travel, especially air travel, which is dehydrating. Hydrosols are also refreshing in the car — try using them to enliven your daily commute. They are also perfect for those of us living in drier climates, which tend to dehydrate the skin.

Hydrosols can also be used in making perfume, eau de cologne, and toilet water.

Hydrosol Blends

I created the following hydrosol blends while working in a skin clinic. They're the result of my own observation and study of the French concepts of skin care and hydrosol blending.

Velleda

1 ounce Roman chamomile hydrosol
1 ounce rose geranium hydrosol
2 ounces Bulgarian rose hydrosol

Mix all ingredients in a 4-ounce plastic spray bottle and shake well. **To use:** Misting the face and neck with this blend works to refresh your spirit and rejuvenate your skin on a deep cellular level. The effect is more profound with mature or aging skin. It is also good for very sensitive skin and imparts a natural glow.

Hydra

1 ounce neroli hydrosol
1 ounce rosemary hydrosol
2 ounces French lavender hydrosol

Mix all ingredients in a 4-ounce plastic spray bottle and shake to create a rare and beautiful water solution. **To use:** This blend is lovely for both the skin and the psyche; it rejuvenates the mind and maintains skin freshness if you live in a dry climate.

Naiad

1 tablespoon lemon verbena hydrosol
1 ounce sweet thyme hydrosol
2 ounces lavender hydrosol

Mix all ingredients in a 4-ounce plastic spray bottle and shake. **To use:** Naiad is useful for overactive sebaceous glands, blemishes, acne, and problem skin types.

Delphi

1 ounce rose geranium hydrosol
2 ounces lavender hydrosol

Mix all ingredients in a 4-ounce plastic spray bottle and shake. **To use:** This blend is energizing, a fast pick-me-up when you need to perform at your best. It also rejuvenates the skin.

Rejuvenating Blend

1 part rose geranium hydrosol
1 part rosemary hydrosol

Mix all ingredients in a plastic spray bottle and shake.

Soothing Blend

1 part lavender hydrosol
1 part thyme hydrosol

Mix all ingredients in a plastic spray bottle and shake.

Water Therapy

Balneotherapy is the art of water therapy, and it is one of aromatherapy's best friends. There is nothing quite so soothing and relaxing as a leisurely soak in a hot bath. As the warmth of the water cradles your physical body, providing relief from the constant pull of gravity, your psyche is refreshed and restored, the weight of the world momentarily lifted. Add a few drops of well-selected essential oils, and you approach nirvana.

Water is nature's greatest and most effective solvent. It acts as a liquid suspension, carrying a variety of minerals and chemicals, depending on its source. When we immerse our bodies in a warm bath, our skin rapidly begins to absorb chemicals that are suspended in the water. These chemical components can make their way to our bloodstream in as little as 2 to 15 minutes. It will take a normally healthy person 30 minutes to 3 hours to eliminate most of these chemicals through the expired breath and urine. In unhealthy or obese people, this process may take up to

10 hours. That is why adding essential oils to a bath is such an effective aromatherapy treatment.

Balneotherapy is built on this solvency. Just as we absorb the essential oils we intentionally add to the water, we absorb a variety of other chemicals and minerals suspended in the water. No two waters are exactly the same. Spring-waters, often thought of as pure, actually contain a variety of minerals. It is the presence of these minerals, from the depths of the earth, that makes certain springwaters highly valued for their curative properties.

Aromatherapy Baths

You can create your own spa experience with just a few oils and a tub of hot water. An aromatherapy bath is the ulti-mate luxury. Experiment with 3 to 5 drops of several com-plementary oils, adjusting the total amount to suit your individual taste. You can add the oils directly to the bath or, for added luxury, disperse them in a cup of milk first. In the list that follows, you'll find combinations of essential oils that you might try for the bath.

• **Soothe Your Worries Away:** lavender, chamomile, and geranium

• **Floral Escape:** rose, bois de rose, and yang-ylang

• **Pampered and Scented:** bois de rose, frankincense, clary sage, and geranium

• **Deep Forest Pool:** pine, rosemary, and eucalyptus

 Other Bath Additives

Essential oils combine well with all other bath additives. Try adding any of the following to your aromatherapy bath:

• Epsom salts, sea salts, and algae to mineralize the water and increase buoyancy

• Oatmeal or honey to soothe and nourish the skin

• Bicarbonate of soda to "soften" the water

• Fresh or dried herbs and flower petals for their aesthetic and therapeutic qualities

- **Luxurious Soak:** Roman chamomile, angelica, neroli, and clary sage
- **Escape to the Woods:** sandalwood, neroli, and cedarwood
- **Vitality:** ravensara, thyme, and MQV
- **Very Calm Night Soak:** marjoram, cypress, and lavender

Aromatherapeutic Milk Bath

Try this version of Cleopatra's famous bathing ritual and see if your skin doesn't feel softer and smoother.

    1 cup instant, powdered whole goat's or cow's milk
    1 tablespoon apricot kernel, jojoba, avocado, hazelnut, or
      extra-virgin olive oil
    8 drops essential oil of German or Roman chamomile, laven-
      der, rosemary, spearmint, or rose

Pour the powdered milk and apricot kernel, jojoba, avocado, hazelnut, or olive oil together directly under running bathwater. Add the essential oil immediately before you step into the tub. Swish with your hands to mix. Now relax!

Make Your Own Bath & Massage Oils

Bath and massage oils are very easy to make at home. You simply need a base oil and any essential oil you desire. I like to use jojoba oil as my base because it does not need refrigeration and will not go rancid. Grapeseed, apricot kernel, and hazelnut oils also make great base oils because they are very light, but they must be refrigerated.

Uplifting, Energizing Oil

- 1 tablespoon jojoba oil
- 2 drops eucalyptus essential oil
- 2 drops peppermint essential oil
- 2 drops rosemary essential oil

Combine all ingredients. Add to your bath while the tap is running to mix well. For a deodorizing foot treatment, have a friend massage your clean, tired feet with the oil for 15 minutes Then put on socks, and go to bed.

Exotic Oil

Pamper yourself outrageously with this luxurious formula. Added to a warm bath, it conditions dry skin and leaves it inbued with a sensual, musky fragrance. Perfect for a cold winter night or a special occasion.

- ¾ cup jojoba oil
- ¼ teaspoon sandalwood essential oil
- ¼ teaspoon patchouli essential oil
- ¼ teaspoon vetiver essential oil
- ¼ teaspoon synthetic musk oil (optional)

Mix all ingredients, adding the musk oil last. Store the blend away from heat and light in a tightly sealed, 8-ounce, dark glass bottle. **To use:** Add 2 teaspoons of the blend to your bath while the tub is filling. Sit back and enjoy!

Nourishing Oil

This vitamin- and mineral-rich formula is good for all skin types, especially normal and dry. Excellent for dry, ragged cuticles, too.

1 tablespoon almond oil
1 tablespoon apricot kernel oil
1 tablespoon avocado oil
1 tablespoon extra-virgin olive oil
1 tablespoon hazelnut oil
1 tablespoon jojoba oil
1,200 international units (IUs) vitamin E oil (d-alpha tocopherol)

Combine all ingredients in an 8-ounce glass or plastic bottle. Tightly cap and shake vigorously. Store in the refrigerator for up to a year. **To use:** For a relaxing and delightfully skin-nourishing bath, add 2 teaspoons of the blend to warm running water. For a delicious and soothing massage, use directly on your skin as needed.

Aromatherapy Massage

A well-selected essential oil formula enhances any type of massage or bodywork. There are many great books on massage, and hands-on courses are available in most major cities. I believe massage is best learned and practiced with another person. You can glean a lot of practical information from reading about it, but you need to feel and touch to really develop massage techniques. If you are inexperienced and feel insecure about giving or receiving a massage, I have included some tips to help you. Whatever the level of your massage training, aromatherapy can be added. By including essential oils, you will enhance the pleasure and benefits of the treatment.

 Fatigue

Rosemary makes a great massage oil for fatigue, and it blends well with lavender and geranium. You must dilute rosemary oil before applying to the skin. Add 20 drops to 1 ounce of carrier oil, or add 15 to 20 drops to bathwater.

When using essential oils in a massage treatment, choose oils that the person receiving the massage finds agreeable to smell. If you experiment with your own blends, keep in mind that a 2 to 4 percent solution (7 to 20 drops of essential oil to 1 ounce of carrier oil) usually makes an appropriate concentration for a massage oil. Limit your blends to no more than three or four different essential oils. One ounce of oil is more than enough for a massage, unless you are massaging a very large, dry, muscular, or hairy person.

 Soreness

To ease the pain of muscle cramps, sore tendons, arthritis, or overexertion in general, the clean, fresh, lemony scent of essential oil of *Eucalyptus citriodora* makes a soothing addition to massage oil. Add 10 to 15 drops of essential oil to ½ cup of almond, hazelnut, grapeseed, or soybean oil, mix well, and massage away the discomfort. Enlist the help of a partner or good friend if possible, and promise to return the favor.

Essential Oils for De-Stressing

There are numerous ways to choose essential oils for massage. Because massage is such an effective way of transcending emotional barriers, I like to choose massage oils for their psychological effects.

Emotional Challenge	Essential Oils to Aid the Process
Anger (to soothe)	Chamomile, ylang-ylang
Anger (unexpressed)	Rosemary
Anxiety	Bergamot, citrus oils, melissa
Depression	Clary sage, bergamot, jasmine
Suicidal tendencies	Clary sage
Insomnia	Marjoram, neroli
Digestive trouble	Fennel, peppermint, cinnamon
Fear	Geranium, juniper, hyssop
Loss	Cypress, ud (agarwood), spikenard
Mental stress	Basil, citrus oils, neroli
Need for calming	Sandalwood, lemongrass, lavender
Physical pain	Ylang-ylang, clary sage, birch, spikenard
Oversensitivity	Mimosa, bois de rose
Need for spiritual, psychic protection	Frankincense, yarrow
Stress	Lavender, geranium, bergamot

Some Basic Massage Tips

• Make sure that the room is a comfortable temperature. A warm, well-ventilated room is preferable. Soft background music and low lights or candlelight can greatly enhance the atmosphere.

• Find a still point within yourself before you begin. Start by centering yourself, breathing evenly and deliberately. Feel your energy as it rises through your body, from your feet to your fingertips.

• Start slowly, using gentle, long, smooth, connecting strokes.

• Pay attention to muscle knots, constricted breathing, and soft sighs. Take note of tender or painful spots as well as pleasure sites.

• Refrain from chatter. Follow your recipient's lead in conversation and don't be offended if he or she doesn't talk at all

Aroma Points and Meridians

Electromagnetic nerve channels run all through the human body. The energy of life, known in the East as *chi* or *qi*, runs along these channels. Although chi is difficult to explain, it is real and can be felt. I have felt chi come through my hands while practicing Tai Chi. I have felt it shoot up my spine during deep yoga practice. The concept of this unseen and immeasurable energy, while new to Western culture, has ruled Eastern thought for many centuries. Acupuncture treatments work from a knowledge of chi and its pathways.

The Chinese say that chi comes into the body with the breath, then flows through twelve paired channels called *meridians*. These meridians can become blocked, and excess heat or cold can deplete or cause excess energy. Through pulse diagnosis, these patterns can be understood. Symptoms are seen as specific expressions of an organ meridian's state of balance or imbalance. The acupuncturist's task is to rebalance the chi.

Volatile in nature and electromagnetic in composition, essential oils have important, subtle psychological and physiological properties. If you accept the concept of chi and acknowledge the healing power of essential oils, it is clear that essential oils influence the chi. Through study, conjecture, intuition, and practice, I have identified some specific oils that have a balancing effect on the organ meridians.

I have also explored chi pulse correlations to specific patterns in music. For example, musical chords in A major and B major influence the gallbladder and liver meridians. The growing awareness and acceptance of vibrational medicine opens an exciting realm of possibility in the relationships of scent, sound, color, and the meridians.

The diagrams on the facing page show the location of meridian points (indicated by black dots) used in traditional Chinese medicine practices of acupressure and acupuncture to stimulate and balance energy flow in corresponding areas of the body. Applying massage oils to these points can be beneficial as well.

Meridian Points

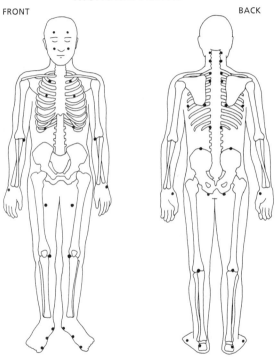

There are numerous acupressure meridians on the face. The gallbladder meridian starts at the outside corner of the eye, winds around the ear, and runs down the side of the head, tracing a shape like that of a Greek war helmet. Sinus and allergy problems originate here, and balancing this meridian can clear the sinuses and the eyes.

The stomach meridian runs through the center of the cheek and nose area, all the way down to the feet. Dry lips and a stuffy, sometimes bloody nose are indications that the stomach meridian is out of balance. Some TMJ problems can be helped by balancing this meridian.

The bladder meridian starts at the forehead, near the hairline over each eye, and runs straight back over the crown of the head to the nape of the neck. It continues down the back, where it splits into two forks that run all the way down each side of the spine.

The small intestine meridian runs along the smile line, from the corner of the nose down to the chin. Breakouts and rashes along this line can indicate food allergies and digestive or eliminative problems.

Other meridians, such as the heart/kidney and spleen/liver, show up on the hands and feet instead of the face. However, all organs are represented on the tongue, in the iris of the eye, and in the ear points.

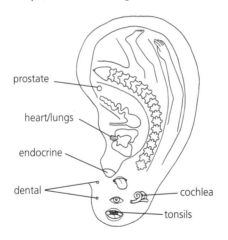

prostate

heart/lungs

endocrine

dental

cochlea

tonsils

Meridians on the ear correspond to various organs and body parts.

Reflexology Points of the Feet

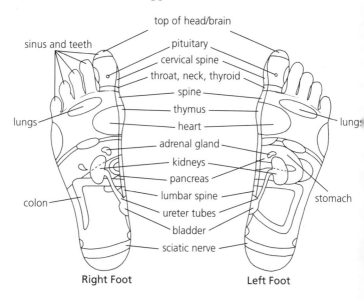

According to reflexology theory, points on the hands and feet stimulate corresponding body parts, as noted in the diagrams on this page and the facing page.

Reflexology Points of the Hands

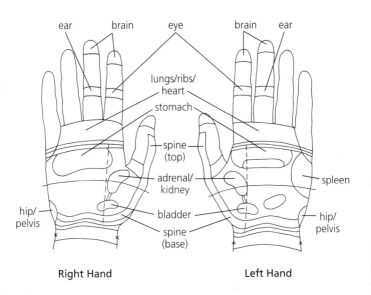

Right Hand

Left Hand

Aromatherapy for Major Organ Meridians and Corresponding Emotions

Organ Meridian	Essential Oils*
Lung/Large Intestine	Eucalyptus, inula, peppermint, pine
Heart/Small Intestine	Anise, lemon verbena, melissa, rose, ylang-ylang
Stomach/Spleen	Dill, fennel, kewda, Roman chamomile
Gallbladder/Liver	Lemon, neroli, peppermint, rosemary, rosemary 'verbenon'
Kidney/Bladder	Cedarwood, geranium, juniper, sandalwood
Umbilicus/Diaphragm	Frankincense, inula, lavender, spikenard, ud

*Use singly diluted or in combination of 2 or 3 oils.

Emotions/Attitudes

Grief and sadness. Possessiveness is the principal cause of grief and results in all kinds of accumulations, such as cysts and tumors.

Trying too hard, pretending you're okay when you're really not. You don't grow old from laughing! Joy is the positive side of all emotions.

Fear. Where fear exists, love is absent. Where love exists, there is no fear.

Worry is payment on a debt never owed. Obsession, thinking too much, overanalyzing.

Anger, resentment, bitter frustration. Encourages compassion and understanding. A deep laugh helps release anger and fears.

A combination of all emotions. Fear of death.

Other Storey Titles You Will Enjoy

The Aromatherapy Companion, by Victoria H. Edwards. This comprehensive aromatherapy guide includes profiles of essential oils and gives instructions for using them in a wide range of recipes for beauty, health, and well-being. 288 pages. Paperback. ISBN 1-58017-150-8.

The Essential Oils Book, by Colleen K. Dodt. This practical guide shows how essential oils can greatly improve the quality of busy lives. Contains dozens of recipes for combating stress, PMS, sunburn, and other common conditions. Comprehensive coverage includes information on which essential oils to use regularly, which to use with caution, and which to avoid altogether. 160 pages. Paperback. ISBN 0-88266-913-3.

The Healing Aromatherapy Bath, by Margo Valentine Lazzara. Combine easy-to-find pure essential oils with simple visualization and meditation techniques to create healing baths specially formulated to address your every mood and need. 160 pages. Paperback. ISBN 1-58017-197-4.

These books and other Storey books are available at
your bookstore, farm store, garden center, or directly from
Storey Books, 210 Mass MoCA Way, North Adams, MA 01247,
or by calling 1-800-441-5700. Or visit our Web site at www.storey.com.